2024 edition Chair Yoga For Seniors Over 60

Gentle stretches for a Healthier Golden Age

Table of Content

Introduction

"As we journey through life, our bodies undergo natural transformations that can affect our balance, flexibility, and mobility. After 60, health conditions like arthritis or stiffness may limit our physical abilities. But what if you could regain flexibility, confidence, and body control from the comfort of your own chair? Chair yoga offers a gentle, modified approach to traditional yoga, adapting poses to accommodate mobility limitations and physical needs. With the support and stability of a chair, you can:

- Restore flexibility and range of motion
- Build confidence and balance
- Regain control over your body
- Enjoy a more active and healthy life

All from the comfort and safety of your own chair!"

"Welcome to Chair Yoga! This book is designed to guide you through a progressive journey, starting with foundational poses and gradually advancing to more challenging routines. To get the most out of this book:

1. Start slow: Begin with the introductory poses and gradually increase your practice as you become more comfortable.
2. Follow the sequences*: Each routine is carefully designed to build upon previous poses, so follow the sequences to maximize the benefits..
3. Listen to your body: Honor your physical limitations and take breaks when needed.
4. Practice regularly*: Consistency is key to experiencing progress and enjoying the full benefits of chair yoga.
5. Use the chair for support: Don't be afraid to rely on the chair for stability and balance – it's there to help you build confidence and strength.

By following these guidelines, you'll be able to maximize the benefits of this book and enjoy a

Embark on a journey towards improved health, heightened vitality, and a more balanced mental state by introducing chair yoga into your life. Together, let's embark on this amazing journey!

CHAPTER 1

Understanding Chair Yoga

1. What is Chair Yoga?

Chair yoga is a modified and adaptive form of yoga that makes the practice accessible to everyone, regardless of mobility or flexibility limitations. By using a chair for support and stability, individuals with restricted mobility, balance concerns, or difficulty getting on and off the floor can experience the benefits of yoga. Chair yoga maintains the core principles of traditional yoga, focusing on mindfulness, breath control, and gentle movements to promote both mental and physical wellbeing. This approach empowers individuals to cultivate strength, flexibility, and balance in a safe and supportive environment."

History and Origins

"Yoga has a rich history spanning thousands of years, originating in ancient India. Traditional yoga aims to harmonize body, mind, and spirit through a diverse range of postures, breathing techniques, and meditation practices. As yoga spread globally, its evolution led to the development of chair yoga - a modified and adaptive approach that makes this ancient practice accessible to diverse populations. This innovative adaptation enables individuals who may have previously faced barriers, such as the elderly and those with physical disabilities, to experience the numerous benefits of yoga. By bridging the gap between traditional yoga and modern needs, chair yoga has opened doors to a more inclusive and supportive practice, fostering wellness and spiritual growth for all."

Key Principles of Chair Yoga

1. Adaptability: Chair yoga adapts poses to meet individual needs and abilities, using props like blocks, belts, and chairs to support and enhance the practice.
2. Breath Awareness: Mindful breathing is a core element, promoting relaxation,

reducing stress, and deepening body-mind connection.

3. Mindfulness: Chair yoga encourages present-moment awareness, fostering inner peace and self-awareness.
4. Safety:Prioritizing safe alignment and modification, chair yoga ensures a injury-free and therapeutic practice.
5. Inclusivity: Accessible to all, regardless of age, physical ability, or fitness level, chair yoga welcomes everyone to experience its benefits.

These principles embody the essence of chair yoga, emphasizing adaptability, mindful breathing, mindfulness, safety, and inclusivity.

By understanding these principles, you'll be better prepared to embark on your chair yoga journey. In the following chapters, you'll learn how to get started with chair yoga, explore various poses, and discover how to tailor your practice to your individual needs and goals.

Chapter 2

Getting Started

Choosing the Right Chair

Choosing the right chair is essential for a safe and effective chair yoga practice. When selecting a chair, consider the following key characteristics:

1. Sturdy and Stable: Ensure the chair is stable and doesn't wobble. Avoid chairs with wheels unless they are lockable.
2. No Armrests: Chairs without armrests provide a greater range of motion for various postures.
3. Firm and Level Seating: Opt for a firm, level seat. While padded chairs are acceptable, avoid seats that are too soft or sloping.
4. Ideal Height: Choose a chair that allows your knees to be at a 90-degree angle, with your feet flat on the ground

By selecting a chair that meets these criteria, you'll be well on your way to a comfortable and effective chair yoga practic

Safety Precautions

The most important thing when doing chair yoga is safety. To guarantee a safe practice, adhere to these guidelines:

1. Make Clear Space: Ensure that there is adequate room to move around your chair without encountering any obstructions.
2. Wear Loose, Comfortable Clothes: Opt for clothing that is relaxed and allows for effortless movement.
3. Pay Attention to Your Body: Proceed cautiously and gently. Stop and modify your

posture or move on to another pose if you experience any pain or discomfort.

4. Use Props: To enhance your practice and make poses more accessible, make use of yoga props like straps, blocks, and cushions.

Keep water close by and take breaks as needed to stay hydrated.

Essential Equipment and Accessories

Chair yoga doesn't require a lot of equipment, but having the following things can help you practice better

1. Yoga Mat: To stop slippage and give your feet some padding, place a yoga mat below your chair.
2. Yoga Strap: In some poses, using a strap can aid with alignment and flexibility.
3. Yoga Blocks: These can be used to adjust positions and make them more accessible while also offering support.

Use blankets and cushions to enhance your comfort and support, particularly when you're relaxing and in seated poses.

Establishing a secure and cozy space and utilizing the appropriate tools will lay the groundwork for an effective chair yoga practice. You will be guided by the following chapters as you master the fundamental poses, get ready for your practice, and progressively improve your abilities.

Chapter 3

Preparing for Your Practice

Creating a Comfortable Space

Having a designated, clutter-free area can improve your chair yoga practice. Here's how to prepare your space for practice:

1. Quiet Environment: Choose a quiet spot free from distractions. This fosters a serene and concentrated environment.
2. Sufficient Lighting: Make sure the area is adequately illuminated. While natural light

is best, a calm atmosphere can also be produced using gentle, ambient lighting.

3. Appropriate Ventilation: Enough air movement is critical. To maintain adequate ventilation, open the windows or turn on the fan, make sure the room is at a suitable temperature—neither too hot nor too cold.
4. Personal Touches: To make a room feel tranquil and welcoming, add accessories like a potted plant, essential oils, or a playlist of soothing music.

Warm-Up Exercises

In order to prepare your body for chair yoga, you must warm up. Here are some easy workouts to get you going:

1. Neck Rolls: Take a tall seated position, bring your chin up to your chest, and slowly move your head side to side.
2. Shoulder shrugs: Raise your shoulders to your ears and then lower and lower them again.
3. Arm Circles: Raise your arms to the sides and slowly widen the circles you make.
4. Marching while seated: Raise one knee at a time to mimic a marching motion.

Rotate your ankles in circles by lifting one foot off the ground and then switching to the other foot.

A fundamental aspect of yoga is pranayama, or breath control. By using these methods, you can improve your yoga practice and promote mental calmness:

1. Deep Breathing: As you sit up straight and put your hands on your stomach, slowly inhale deeply through your nose, feeling your tummy rise. Breathe out through your mouth while feeling your stomach drop.
2. Using the alternate nostril breathing method: cover your right nostril with your thumb, breathe in through your left nostril, shut it with your right ring finger, and then release the breath through your right nostril. Continue on the opposite side.
3. Box breathing involves inhaling for four counts, holding your breath for four counts, exhaling for four counts, and then holding it for an additional four counts. Repeat many times.
4. Lion's Breath: Take a deep breath through your nose, spread your lips, stretch your tongue out, and then let out a forceful "ha" sound as you exhale.

You'll be ready to start your chair yoga practice by setting up your area, getting your body warm, and engaging in mindful breathing. The upcoming chapters will walk you through chair yoga postures that are basic, intermediate, and advanced, assisting you in creating a complete and pleasurable practice.

Chapter 4

Seated Mountain Pose (Tadasana)

How to Do It: Take a straight seat and place your feet hip-width apart on the floor. Your hands should be by your sides or on your thighs. Activate your core, extend your spine, and roll your shoulders back and down.

- Advantages: Enhances body awareness, develops core muscles, and improves posture.

Seated Cat-Cow Stretch

(Marjaryasana-Bitilasana)

Putting your hands on your knees is how to do it. Bend your back, raise your chest, and raise your gaze while inhaling (Cow Pose). Exhale, curve your back, bring your chin to your chest, and lower yourself into the cat pose. Repeat many times.

Benefits: Releases stress, stretches the neck and back, and improves spine flexibility.

Forward Bend While Seated (Paschimottanasana)

How to Do It: Place your feet hip-width apart and sit on the edge of your chair. Take a breath and stretch your back. Take a breath out, bend forward at the hips, and extend your hands to your shins or the ground.

Benefits: Relaxes the mind and stretches the shoulders, hamstrings, and back.

Seated Spinal Twist (Ardha Matsyendrasana)

How to Do It: With your feet flat on the ground, sit sideways in your chair. Using both hands, grasp the rear of the chair. Exhale and twist your torso towards the back of the chair after taking a breath and lengthening your spine. After a few breaths of holding, switch sides.

Benefits: Promotes better digestion, eases back strain, and increases spinal mobility.

Seated Hip Opener (Agni Stambhasana)

How to Do It: Sit with your feet flat on the floor. Put your left knee over your right ankle. To save your knee, flex your right foot. As you sit up straight, use your right hand to gently press your right knee down. After a few breaths of holding, switch sides.

Benefits: Increases hip flexibility and stretches the lower back, glutes, and hips.

Seated Shoulder Stretch

Sit with your feet flat on the ground to do the action. Raise your right arm to shoulder height and spread it across your body. Press your right arm gently toward your chest with your left hand. After a few breaths of holding, switch sides.

Benefits: Increases flexibility, releases tension, and stretches the upper back and shoulders.

Side Stretch While Seated

Sit with your feet flat on the ground to do the action. Feel a stretch down your right side as you lift your right arm above your head and slant to the left. After a few breaths of holding, switch sides.

Benefits: Releases tension, increases flexibility, and stretches the body's sides.

Seated Ankle to Knee Pose (Eka Pada Rajakapotasana Variation)

Sit with your feet flat on the ground to do the action. Form a figure-four by placing your right ankle on top of your left knee. Bend your right foot and use your right hand to gently press down on your right knee. After a few breaths of holding, switch sides.

Benefits: Increases hip flexibility, opens the hips, and stretches the lower back and glutes.

Seated Knee to Chest Pose (Apanasana)

Sit with your feet flat on the ground to do the action. Raise your right knee to your chest and give it a firm squeeze with both hands.

Take a few deep breaths and sit up straight. Change positions.

Benefits: Promotes better digestion; stretches the thighs, hips, and lower back.

You'll establish a solid foundation for your practice by becoming proficient in these fundamental chair yoga positions. More intermediate and advanced poses will be covered in the upcoming chapters to help you improve your flexibility, strength, and general health.

Chapter 5

Intermediate Chair Yoga Poses

Seated Warrior Pose (Virabhadrasana)

How to Do It: Sit sideways on your chair, place your foot flat on the floor, and bend your right leg to a 90-degree angle behind you. Lift your arms up and turn your palms towards one another. After holding for a few breaths, switch sides.

Benefits: Enhances balance and endurance, strengthens the legs and core.

Seated Side Stretch (Parighasana)

Sit with your feet flat on the ground to do the action. While keeping your left foot flat on the ground, extend your right leg to the side. Take a breath, lift your right arm above your head, bend to the left, and reach for your left foot. After holding for a few breaths, switch sides.

Benefits: Opens the hips, increases flexibility, and stretches the sides of the body.

Seated Sun Salutations (Surya Namaskar)

Steps to Take: Lie back with your feet flat on the ground. Take a breath, lift your arms above your head, and lift your gaze upward.

Take a breath out, bend forward, and reach for the ground.

Taking a deep breath, bend your knees, arch your back, and gaze upwards, assuming the cow pose.

Exhale, round your spine and tuck your chin (Cat Pose).

Breathe in and raise your arms aloft once again.

Let go and bring your arms down to your sides.

Benefits: Boosts circulation, increases flexibility, and gives the body energy.

Seated Eagle Pose (Garudasana)

Method: Assume a tall posture and place your feet flat on the ground. If at all feasible, wrap your right foot around your left leg and cross your right thigh over your left thigh. Bring your hands together and cross your left arm across your right at the elbows. While maintaining a downward posture, raise your elbows and fingertips. After holding for a few breaths, switch sides.

Benefits: Enhances focus and balance; stretches the hips, upper back, and shoulders.

Seated Pigeon Pose (Kapotasana)

Sit with your feet flat on the ground to do the action. Form a figure-four by placing your right ankle on top of your left knee. Bend your right foot and use your right hand to gently press down on your right knee. Lean forward a little bit if it's comfortable to increase the stretch. After holding for a few breaths, switch sides.

Benefits: Increases hip flexibility, opens the hips, and stretches the lower back and glutes.

Seated Chair Pose (Utkatasana)

How to Do It: Place your feet hip-width apart and sit on the edge of your chair. Breathe in, extend your arms overhead, then release the breath as you flex your hips slightly forward while maintaining a straight back and using your core. Take several deep breaths and hold.

Benefits: Enhances posture and balance; strengthens the glutes, thighs, and core.

Boat Pose in Sitting (Navasana)

How to Do It: Place your feet flat on the ground and sit on the edge of your chair. For support, grasp the chair's sides. Raise your feet off the ground, tighten your core, and slant your knees toward your chest. If you can, raise your arms in front of you. Take several deep breaths and hold.

Benefits: Increases attention, balance, and core strength.

Seated Camel Pose (Ustrasana)

Method: Assume a tall posture and place your feet flat on the ground. With your fingers pointed down, place your hands on your lower back. Taking a deep breath, raise your chest and slightly arch your back while gazing upward at the ceiling. Take several deep breaths and hold.

Benefits: Increases spinal flexibility, opens the shoulders and chest, and stretches the front of the body.

Through the integration of these intermediate poses into your routine, you'll enhance your strength, flexibility, and stability. To assist you develop further into your practice, the upcoming chapters will introduce you to increasingly challenging positions and whole chair yoga sequences.

Chapter 6

Advanced Chair Yoga Poses

☐ Balance Pose

How to Do It: Place your feet flat on the ground and sit on the edge of your chair. For support, grasp the chair's sides. Raise your feet off the ground, contract your core, and slant your back slightly. Maintaining a straight back, extend your legs forward. Take several deep breaths and hold.

Benefits: Increases stability and balance; strengthens the core.

Seated Tree Pose (Vrksasana)

Method: Assume a tall posture and place your feet flat on the ground. Put your right foot—not your knee—on your inner left thigh or calf. Raise your arms above your head or firmly press your hands together at your chest. After holding for a few breaths, switch sides.

Benefits include increased attention, stronger legs and core, and improved balance.

Seated Bridge Pose (Setu Bandhasana)

How to Do It: Place your feet flat on the ground and sit on the edge of your chair. For support, grasp the chair's sides. Using your core and glutes, raise your hips off the chair. Keep your back straight and your feet firmly planted. Take several deep breaths and hold.

Benefits: Increases spinal flexibility and strengthens the hamstrings, glutes, and back.

Chair Yoga Flow Sequences

Flow Sequence 1: Energizing Flow

Start with a few deep breaths in the seated mountain pose.

Seated Cat-Cow Stretch: Move through 5-6 rounds.

Do three to four cycles of Sun Salutations while seated.

Hold each side for a few breaths while in the seated warrior pose.

Hold each side for a few breaths while in the seated Eagle Pose.

Stretching while seated: Take a few breaths to hold each side.

Flow Sequence 2: Relaxing Flow

Bend forward while seated and hold for a few breaths.

Hold each side of the seated spinal twist for a few breaths.

Hold each side for a few breaths during the seated hip opener.

Take a few breaths and hold each side of the seated shoulder stretch.

Hold each side for a few breaths while in the seated knee to chest pose.

Seated Meditation: Close your eyes and sit quietly while concentrating on taking slow, deep breaths.

Flow Sequence 3: Strengthening Flow

Hold the seated chair pose for a few breaths.

Hold the chair balance pose for a few breaths.

Hold for a few breaths in the seated boat pose.

Hold each side for a few breaths while in the seated tree pose.

Hold for a few breaths in the seated bridge pose.

Hold the chair balance pose for a few breaths.

Blending Flows

You are welcome to mix and match parts of the various sequences to build a practice that is specific to your needs and level of energy. Always pay attention to your body's needs and adjust positions as needed to guarantee your comfort and security.

By incorporating these advanced poses and flow sequences into your practice, you'll further enhance your strength, flexibility, and balance. The use of chair yoga for particular medical issues, mental wellbeing, and designing customized routines to fit your lifestyle are all covered in the upcoming chapters.

Chapter 7

Chair Yoga for Specific Health Conditions

Chair Yoga for Arthritis

Focus: Mild motions to enhance joint mobility and lessen stiffness.

Pose:

The seated mountain pose develops the muscles and helps with posture.

Flexibility in the spine is increased and stiffness is decreased with the seated cat-cow stretch.

Improves spinal mobility and facilitates digestion with the Seated Spinal Twist.

Lower back and hip tension is released in the seated knee to chest pose.

Chair Yoga for Back Pain

Focus: To reduce pain, stretch your back and strengthen your core.

Pose:

Seated forward bends target the hamstrings and back, promoting flexibility. The Seated Spinal Twist enhances spinal flexibility and alleviates tension. The Seated Cat-Cow Stretch strengthens and expands the back muscles. Additionally, seated hip openers effectively release tension in the hips and lower back, promoting relaxation and mobility."

Yoga for Osteoporosis

The main goals are to strengthen bones and enhance balance to avoid falls.

Pose:

"Seated Warrior Pose builds strength in the legs and improves balance. The seated Tree Pose enhances stability and balance. The seated Bridge Pose strengthens the hips and back, while seated side stretches increase flexibility and expand the chest. These poses, adapted for seated practice, promote strength, balance, and flexibility."!

Chair Yoga for Diabetes

Goals: Increasing blood flow and lowering tension.

Pose:

"Seated Sun Salutations stimulate circulation, boosting energy levels. Seated forward bends promote circulation and mental serenity. Seated Spinal Twists support digestive health and detoxification. The Seated Knee to Chest Pose stretches the lower back, improves circulation, and enhances overall well-being. These seated adaptations of traditional yoga poses offer numerous physical and mental health benefits."

Chair Yoga for Heart Health

Focus: Moderate exercise to lower stress and enhance cardiovascular health.

Pose:

"The Seated Mountain Pose engages the core, promoting strong posture and stability. Seated shoulder stretches release tension and relax the upper body. Seated side stretches enhance flexibility and expand the chest. Additionally, Seated Breathing Techniques reduce stress and anxiety, improving lung capacity and overall well-being. These seated yoga poses and breathing techniques offer a holistic approach to physical and mental wellness."

Chair Yoga for Anxiety and Stress Relief

Focus: Mindfulness and body calming practices for relaxation.

Pose:

"Seated forward bends stretch the back, calming the mind and promoting relaxation. The seated cat-cow stretch reduces stress and anxiety, fostering a sense of calmness. Seated Breathing Techniques feature deep breathing exercises that lower anxiety and promote serenity. Additionally, seated meditation cultivates inner peace, mindfulness, and a sense of inner balance. These practices combine to create a powerful toolkit for managing stress and cultivating overall well-being.

Chair Yoga Enhancing Digestion

Focus: To promote digestion, perform light twists and stretches.

Pose:

"Seated spinal twists stimulate detoxification and enhance digestive function. The seated cat-cow stretch massages the abdominal organs, promoting their health. The seated knee to chest pose alleviates bloating and supports healthy digestion. Additionally, seated forward bends stretch the digestive system, calming the mind and promoting relaxation. These seated yoga poses collectively support overall digestive well-being and promote a sense of calm."

Chair Yoga for Better Sleep

Emphasis: Breathing exercises and calming poses to encourage sound sleep.

Pose:

Benefits of Chair Yoga for Relaxation and Sleep_

1. Seated Forward Bend: Relax the body and mind, promoting overall calmness.
2. Seated Cat-Cow Stretch:Eases stress and encourages relaxation.
3. Seated Breathing Techniques_: Deep breathing exercises prepare the body for sleep.
4. Sitting Meditation: Promotes awareness and prepares the body for restful sleep.

By focusing on these specific health benefits, you can tailor your chair yoga practice to meet your unique needs and goals. In the upcoming chapters, we'll explore the use of chair yoga for mental health, creating customized routines, and incorporating chair yoga into daily activities.

Chapter 8

Chair Yoga for Mental Wellness

Chair Yoga for Stress Relief

Focus: Using attentive breathing and gentle movement to reduce tension.

Pose:

The seated mountain pose helps to create a grounded, peaceful feeling.

Seated Cat-Cow Stretch: This tension-relieving exercise combines movement and breathing.

Bending forward while seated: Encourages calmness and reduces tension.

Deep, slow breathing exercises are a useful way to lower stress levels when seated.

Chair Yoga for Anxiety

Focus: Calming the body and mind to reduce anxiety.

Pose:

Relaxes the shoulders and neck with a seated shoulder stretch.

The seated spinal twist helps to alleviate stress and improve balance.

Stretching the body while seated can help to ease anxiety.

Sitting meditation promotes inner calm and mindfulness.

Chair Yoga for Depression

The main goals are to improve wellbeing and mood.

Pose:

Sun Salutations while seated: energise the body and improve mood.

Warrior Pose while Sitting: Increases strength and self-assurance.

Eagle Pose in a sitting position: Promotes concentration and focus.

A reviving and uplifting breathing method is called the "Satisfied Breath of Joy."

Chair Yoga for Cognitive Function

Focus: Improving cognitive performance by focusing and moving mindfully.

Pose:

Tree Pose: Enhances balance and concentration.

Seated Spinal Twist: Enhances mental acuity and nervous system stimulation.

Bending forward while seated: Promotes focus and mental calmness.

Alternate nostril breathing when seated: Promotes mental equilibrium and enhances cognitive performance.

Chair Yoga for Emotional Balance

Focus: Using gentle positions and breathing techniques, achieve emotional harmony.

Pose:

Heart Opener for Sitting: Facilitates emotional release and opens the chest.

Hip flexor strain and stress can be released by sitting in the pigeon pose.

Stretching while seated might help you maintain a flexible and balanced mindset.

Sitting meditation promotes mindfulness and emotional equilibrium.

Chair Yoga for Mindfulness

Focus: Using meditation and yoga practices to cultivate mindfulness.

Pose:

Pose for sitting on a mountain: Promotes grounding and presence.

Breath and focused movement are combined in the Seated Cat-Cow Stretch.

Bending forward while seated: Encourages calm and introspection.

A seated body scan meditation improves mindfulness by guiding consciousness through the body.

Chair Yoga for Energy and Vitality

Focus: Increasing vitality by striking dynamic and energizing positions.

Pose:

Sun Salutations while seated: These invigorate and energise the body.

The seated boat pose improves vitality and strengthens the core.

Chair Balance Pose: Increases vitality and concentration.

Breathing exercise known as the "Sitting Breath of Fire" increases vitality and clarity.

Chair Yoga for Relaxation and Sleep

Focus: Getting the body and mind ready for sound sleep.

Pose:

Bending forward while seated: Relaxes the body and psyche.

The seated cat-cow stretch eases stress and encourages calmness.

Techniques for Seated Breathing: Taking calm, deep breaths may help you get ready for bed.

Sitting meditation promotes calmness and awareness.

Your practice can benefit from these chair yoga poses and mental wellness strategies, which can improve your emotional and mental well-being. The upcoming chapters will walk you through developing customized routines, incorporating chair yoga into everyday activities, and looking into further advice and resources to help you with your practice.

Chapter 9

Creating a Chair Yoga Routine

Setting Your Goals

Identify Your Objectives: Determine what you hope to achieve with your chair yoga practice. Objectives could be controlling particular health concerns, lowering stress, increasing mental clarity, or increasing flexibility.

Make a Strategy: Describe a strategy that supports your objectives. Choose the exact postures or sequences to practice, the number of practice days per week, and the length of each session.

Choosing the Right Poses

Warm-Up Poses: Start with easy poses like Seated Mountain Pose, Seated Cat-Cow Stretch, and Seated Shoulder Shrugs to loosen up your body.

Key Pose: Choose positions that address your objectives. Incorporate the Seated Forward Bend and Seated Spinal Twist for flexibility. Use Seated Warrior and Seated Boat poses to build strength.

Cool-Down postures: Conclude with calming postures like the Seated Forward Bend and Seated Meditation to aid in your body's relaxation.

Structuring Your Routine

Warm-Up (5-10 minutes): Start with gentle stretches and movements to prepare your body.

Example: Seated Mountain Pose, Seated Cat-Cow Stretch, Seated Shoulder Shrugs.

Core Practice (15-25 minutes): Focus on poses that align with your goals.

Example: Seated Warrior Pose, Seated Tree Pose, Seated Pigeon Pose.

Cool-Down (5-10 minutes): Finish with relaxing poses and deep breathing exercises.

Example: Seated Forward Bend, Seated Spinal Twist, Seated Meditation.

Sample Routine for Flexibility

Warm-Up

Chair Yoga Sequence

Warm-Up (2 minutes)

 Seated Mountain Pose

Sequence (14 minutes)

Seated Cat-Cow Stretch (3 minutes)

Core Practice: Seated Forward Bend (3 minutes)

Seated Spinal Twist (3 minutes per side)

 Seated Side Stretch (2 minutes per side)

 Seated Hip Opener (3 minutes per side)

Cool-Down (6 minutes)*

Seated Knee to Chest Pose (3 minutes per side)

This sequence provides a balanced chair yoga practice, covering various aspects of flexibility, strength, and relaxation.

Remember to breathe deeply and smoothly throughout each pose, honoring your body's limitations and comfort. Enjoy the practice!Seated Meditation (5 minutes)

Sample Routine for Strength

Warm-Up:

Seated Mountain Pose (2 minutes)

Seated Shoulder Shrugs (3 minutes)

Core Practice:

Seated Warrior Pose (3 minutes each side)

Seated Boat Pose (3 minutes)

Chair Balance Pose (3 minutes)

Seated Tree Pose (3 minutes each side)

Cool-Down:

Seated Forward Bend (5 minutes)

Seated Breathing Techniques (5 minutes)

Sample Routine for Stress Relief

Warm-Up:

Seated Mountain Pose (2 minutes)

Seated Cat-Cow Stretch (3 minutes)

Core Practice:

Seated Shoulder Stretch (3 minutes each side)

Seated Spinal Twist (3 minutes each side)

Seated Heart Opener (3 minutes)

Seated Side Stretch (3 minutes each side)

Cool-Down:

Seated Forward Bend (5 minutes)

Seated Meditation (5 minutes)

Adjusting Your Routine

Listen to Your Body: Pay attention to how your body feels during and after each session. Modify poses or the duration of your practice as needed to ensure comfort and safety.

Progress Gradually: As you become more comfortable with your practice, gradually increase the duration and intensity of your sessions. Add more challenging poses or longer hold times as appropriate.

Stay Consistent: Regular practice is key to achieving your goals. Aim to practice chair yoga several times a week, even if only for a short duration.

Incorporating Variety

Mix It Up: Change up your routine to prevent boredom. To keep your practice interesting and well-rounded, switch up your positions and patterns.

Examine the Themes: To address different facets of your well-being, concentrate on a different theme every week, such as strength, relaxation, or balance.

Employ props: Use accessories such as straps, blocks, or little weights to improve your technique and provide yourself more support.

Tracking Your Progress

Keep a Practice Journal: Maintain a yoga diary to track your progress toward your goals, log your sessions, and document your feelings both before and after practice.

Honor significant anniversaries: No matter how tiny, recognize and celebrate your accomplishments. Advancements could be in the form of stronger muscles, less stress, or more flexibility.

You can reap the complete benefits of chair yoga by designing a customized regimen that suits your needs and tastes. The upcoming chapters will offer advice on how to include chair yoga into regular activities as well as more resources to help you with your practice.

Chapter 10

Chair Yoga for Daily Activities

Morning Routine

Purpose: Energize your body and mind to start the day with vitality.

An example of a routine

Seated Mountain Pose: To center yourself, sit up straight with your feet flat on the ground. Then, take several deep breaths.

To stimulate circulation and awaken the body, perform three to four cycles of sitting sun salutations.

Stretch your spine gently by performing five to six rounds of the seated cat-cow pose.

Seated Forward Bend: To relax the mind and lengthen the back, hold for a few breaths.

Seated Breathing Techniques: To start the day off well, practice deep breathing for a few minutes.

Work Breaks

Goal: Reduce stress and boost output throughout working hours.

An example of a routine

Seated Shoulder Stretch: To release tension, stretch each shoulder for one to two minutes.

Spinal Twist while Seated: To revitalize your spine, twist to each side for a few breaths.

Seated Side Stretch: To extend your body's sides, hold each position for a minute.

Seated Hip Opener: To relieve tension in the hips, hold each side for one minute.

Seated Meditation: To lower stress and increase attention, practice mindful breathing for two to three minutes.

After Work Routine

Goal: Reduce stress and tension by making the transition from work to relaxation.

An example of a routine

Seated Forward Bend: To relax the mind and lengthen the back, hold for a few breaths.

Perform five to six rounds of the seated cat-cow stretch to release tension in your spine.

Spinal Twist when Seated: To help with digestion and revitalize the spine, twist to either side.

To relieve hip tension, hold each side of the seated pigeon pose for a minute.

Techniques for Deep Breathing While Seated: To relax, practice deep breathing for a few minutes.

Pre-Bedtime Routine

Goal: Get the body and mind ready for a good night's sleep.

An example of a routine

Seated Forward Bend: To relax the body and mind, hold this pose for a few breaths.

To relieve tension, perform five to six rounds of the seated cat-cow stretch.

To ease the lower back and hips, hold each side of the seated knee to chest pose for a minute.

Techniques for Deep, Slow Breathing While Seated: Take deep, slow breaths to be ready for bed.

Seated Meditation: To encourage relaxation, practice attentive meditation for a few minutes.

Including Chair Yoga All Day Long

Stretch at Your Desk: During brief breaks, do easy stretches such as seated forward bends, seated spinal twists, and seated shoulder shrugs.

Take Deep, Slow Breaths to Reduce Stress and Improve Focus: Throughout the day, set aside some time to concentrate on your breathing and practice mindful breathing.

Use Transitions Wisely: Practice brief stretches or postures during transitional periods, such as when you're waiting for a meeting to start or while watching TV commercials.

Integrate Movement: Include mild exercises like sitting leg lifts and raising your arms above your head in your everyday routine.

Customizing Your Routine

Listen to Your Body: To guarantee comfort and safety, pay attention to your body's cues and modify your routine as necessary.

Be Adaptable: Your regimen should be adaptable to allow for fluctuations in your energy or schedule.

Combine Tasks: Combine chair yoga with other everyday routines, such stretching while on the phone or breathing techniques while watching television.

Benefits of Chair Yoga in Daily Life

Increased Flexibility: Maintaining and increasing flexibility via regular practice facilitates smoother and more comfortable daily activities.

Decreased Stress: By lowering stress levels, mindful breathing and movement help to foster peace and wellbeing.

Enhanced Focus: Taking frequent chair yoga breaks might help you be more focused and productive, especially during the workday.

Improved Posture: Regular exercise helps to improve posture, which lowers the risk of neck and back problems.

Enhanced Energy: You can stay active and involved throughout the day by gently moving and breathing deeply.

You may get the advantages of chair yoga throughout the day and improve your general well-being by including this practice into your regular routine. The upcoming chapters will cover more methods to incorporate yoga into your daily life and offer further advice and resources to help you with your chair yoga practice.

Chapter 11

Additional Tips and Resources

Tips for a Successful Chair Yoga Practice

Start Slow: If you're new to yoga, start with easy positions and work your way up to more difficult ones as you gain comfort.

Listen to Your Body: Throughout practice, be aware of how your body feels. If a posture hurts or is uncomfortable for you, pause, adjust, or move on.

Concentrate on Breathing: The secret to a fruitful practice is deep, conscious breathing. Breathe deeply to center yourself and direct your motions.

Remain Consistent: Consistent practice yields greater benefits than infrequent practice. Try to stick to a routine that works for your schedule.

As Needed: Don't be scared to adjust poses to better fit your physical needs. To make it easier for you to get into postures, use props like straps or blocks.

Resources for Chair Yoga

Online Videos: You may follow along with a ton of free chair yoga videos that are available online. Seek out videos suited to your objectives and skill level.

Yoga Apps: A number of applications have been developed expressly for chair yoga, providing instructions on poses and guided routines.

Books: Seek out chair yoga books with thorough directions and posture drawings.

Local courses: For chair yoga courses, inquire at the community centers or yoga studios in your area. If there are no available in-person classes, ask about virtual choices.

Yoga Retreats: To enhance your practice and have a more immersed experience, think about going on a chair yoga retreat.

Incorporating Yoga into Daily Life

Walking Meditation: To engage in mindful walking, concentrate on your breathing, pay attention to each stride, and stay in the present.

Desk Yoga: To relieve stress and sharpen your focus, do some easy stretches and breathing techniques at your desk.

Yoga Nidra: To encourage relaxation and lower stress levels, engage in yoga nidra, also known as yogic slumber. You can do this at a break in your day or right before bed.

Yoga Philosophy: To gain a deeper understanding of yoga that goes beyond the physical postures, study the philosophical parts of the practice, such as the yamas and niyamas.

Community Involvement: To meet people who are interested in yoga and to maintain your practice motivation, join an online group or yoga community.

Conclusion

Incorporating chair yoga into your everyday routine can be easy and accessible while yet offering a host of physical and mental health advantages. Chair yoga has many benefits for your general health; just start off cautiously, pay attention to your body, and practice consistently. Make yoga a regular part of your routine by improving your practice with the help of the offered materials and advice

In conclusion, chair yoga is a versatile and accessible practice that offers a wide range of physical and mental health benefits. Chair yoga can be customized to fit your requirements and lifestyle, whether your goals are to increase flexibility, lower stress, or improve your general well-being.

Chair yoga has many health and life-improving benefits that you can experience if you begin cautiously, pay attention to your body, and practice consistently. Create a customized chair yoga practice that suits you by using the advice, poses, and routines in this book.

Recall that everybody can do chair yoga, regardless of age or degree of fitness. You can enjoy better posture, less stress, more flexibility, and general wellness with consistent practice. So take a seat and begin practicing chair yoga right now!